Beginners Guide To Effective Meditation

Easy Techniques With Tips & Suggestions

I0420541

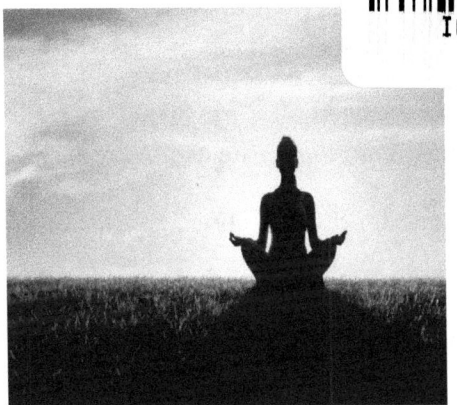

By

Meenakshi Narang

Table of Contents

Beginners guide to effective meditation

2

Chapter 1 - INTRODUCTION

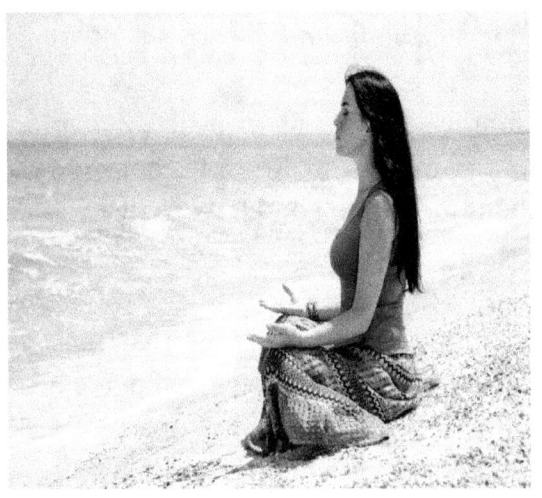

Amidst several types of meditation, meeting a common goal makes meditation suitable to everyone. This book takes you through simple meditation techniques and practices that you can understand and incorporate in your daily lives. This is the best form of relaxation and escape from the stressful lives that we all lead today. This book is going to be ideal those who want to relax their mind and soul with the help of meditation. Understand how these simple practices can have powerful, long-lasting effects on your life.

Embrace the feeling of peace, power and control inside you. Read this book to learn about meditation and how to live a stress free life.

Our mind is like a sponge that saps our experiences. Our feelings and perceptions control the way our mind works. Everyone may not have the ability to understand the mind for its depth. No doubt, this makes our mind confused, and we are unable to deal with day to day stresses.

For a better and a clutter-free living, we must have a better understanding of our minds. Here comes the role of meditation. For excessive stress, utilize meditation to prepare your mind to experience life in its entirety. This will also help in gaining answers to many questions that have been bogging you.

Meditation is the act of training the mind to understand various beneficial states like compassion, understanding, concentration, humility, patience and perseverance. The prime objective of meditation is to relax the mind completely and lay concentration on the internal energy. Meditation can help in regulating the mind to tame down health issues. Some meditation practices involve holding an steady position for several hours. Other practices allow for inculcating that awareness in day to day activities. There may be recitation or chanting of mantras to activate the mind and channelize energy.

At a higher level of mental abilities, people are also able to invoke a certain emotion in order to study and analyze it. Moreover, emotions like anger and hatred can be generated, and a suitable mental response may be cultivated in order to gain control over moods and emotions. Through meditation, you can achieve pure awareness and awake your soul and spirit.

Chapter 2 - Learning Meditation

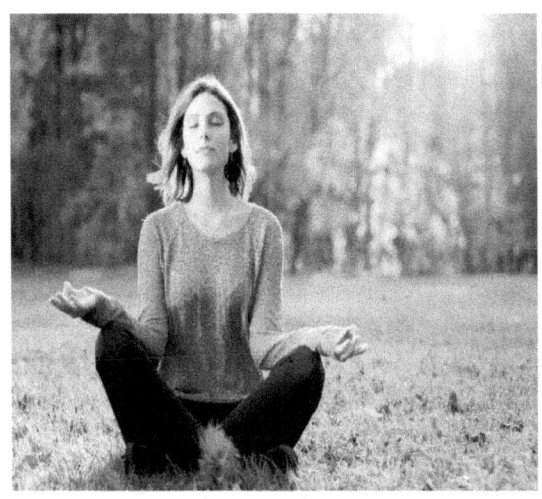

Meditation may seem complex and advanced. However, its techniques and practices have been designed for everyone, especially the beginners. Young or old, all can enjoy the benefits of meditation in a simplified way.

Practice meditation for:
- Relaxing the mind
- Experiencing tranquility anytime and anywhere
- Evoking spiritual energy
- For getting liberation from negative & toxic energies

When you are sleeping and resting your body, your mind continues to work. Even after an entire day of processing different kinds of information, the mind does not rest. Mind also has to deal with things that we fathom such as stress due to work, anger, fear or anxiety. Through meditation, you can focus on the unpleasant and tense state of mind and change attitude towards them. The outcome of this on the different spheres of can be noticed as your practice deepens.

In order to rest your mind, get in touch with all the emotions that we experience. This is possible through meditation. It is just an effort to relax the feelings that can induce negativity. Remember, when you meditate, you do not exactly solve your problems. You only relax your mind and help it deal with any issue easily and rationally.

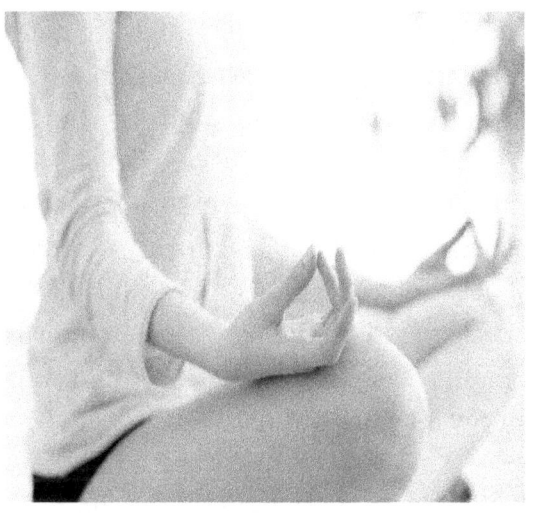

Meditation and its Benefits

There have been several studies on the elements and principles of meditation to create modern methods that can suit our current lifestyles. Meditation is often termed as a seed. Sow this seed; nurture it and it would blossoms. The more it is nurtured, the better it grows and yields. To derive the benefits of meditation one needs to be disciplined and regular with it.

Meditation leads to a change in body's cells infusing them with renewed energy. As a result, an individual is cheerful, fervent and peaceful. It helps in controlling blood pressure, treating insomnia, reducing anxiety attacks, anxiety-related pains like headaches, muscle, and joint pains. This will improve immune system and help in improving energy level in the body.

Healing is promoted during meditation as it initiates the brainwave pattern into an Alpha state, thus, reinvigorates the mind and makes it beautiful.

The benefits of meditation include:

Channelizing of Physical Energy

Meditation helps in channelizing the inherent life energy to your body. This leads to better health. Meditation helps in - controlling high blood pressure; reducing blood lactate levels; reducing anxiety attacks; relieving from headaches, ulcers, muscle and joint problems, and all other conditions that are related to stress; increasing levels of Serotonin to promote better behavior; strengthening of immune system; bettering of energy and enthusiasm levels.

Revitalizing Mental Condition

Practicing meditation techniques renders a longstanding impact on mental health. On exercising your brain continuously, the brain becomes healthier, leading to overall brain functioning. Through meditation, the brainwave pattern can be changed into an alpha state to make the mind healthier and happier.

Some mental benefits of meditation include:

Reduced Anxiety; Improved Emotional Stability; Better Creativity; Increased Happiness; Better Intuition; Clarity and Peace of Mind; Better Focus and Concentration; Expanded Consciousness and Mental Sharpness.

Building Emotional Health

Meditation conditions our mind for positive emotional responses. Negative emotions like anger and depression get replaced by positive and fulfilling emotions. The emotional benefits of meditation include:

- Better insight and moral perspective
- Stress management
- Better self-awareness
- Ability to focus on the present
- Ability to reduce outbursts of negative emotions

Meditation for Personal Growth

Through meditation, you delve deeper into your psychic mind. This gives you a chance actually to embrace your being and discover several wonderful insights into the mystery that life is. With continuous meditation, you can experience the following:

- More understanding of who you are
- Attaining a state of consciousness where you perceive the whole cosmos to be a part of you. This is called the cosmic consciousness.
- This creates a strong flow of love between you and the world.
- Ability to embrace relationships with all the flaws that might exist.

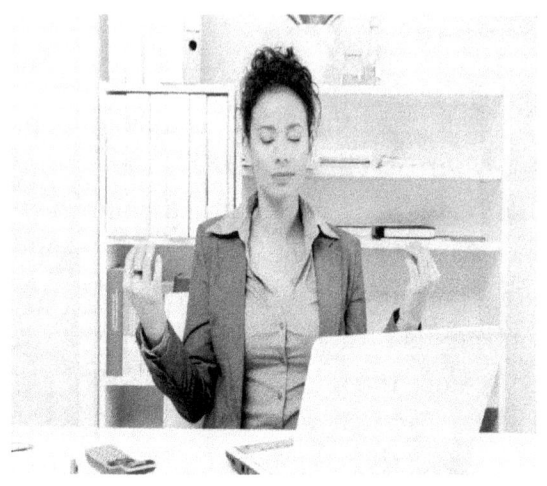

Meditation for Better Performance at Work

When you see a change in your personality and your interaction with the world around you, it is quite natural to experience the change in your workplace.

The benefits of meditation in the work place include:
- More job satisfaction

- Better interpersonal relationships
- Increased performance and efficiency
- More contribution to the progress of the organization
- Ability to stay calm and cope with stress

Chapter 3: Meditate The Right Way

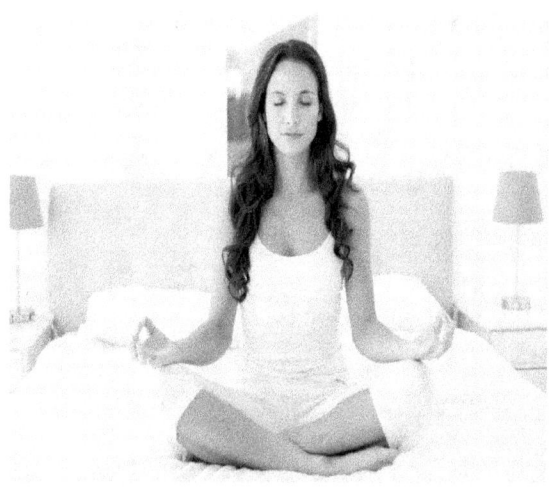

A stressful and an anxious mind is an indication that your mind needs some amount of conditioning. Although meditation might seem just as simple as closing your eyes and focusing your thoughts, in reality, there is a certain way to go about it to get maximum benefits from it.

An essential thing about meditation is to find the right guidance. So, the first step is to find a good teacher who can introduce various techniques that have been passed on through generations. A teacher is essential as he or she has dedicated several years to understand the nuances of meditation. In case you are new to meditation, get the advantage that a teacher will give you to enjoy the benefits of meditation faster. You need not invest too much time in seeking answers from various sources when you have a teacher to guide you through your journey.

Requisites of Meditation

Stay Attentive

Channelize your attention is the first requisite and the most obvious element of meditation. You must be able to focus all your attention to ensure that you are free from all distractions when you are communicating with your inner self.

Simply Relax

Control your breath and it will be easier to focus your attention. By keeping your breathing relaxed and controlled, you will be able to make the most of your meditative time. The technique to get your breathing right is to keep it deep and even. While you do this, be sure to keep the muscles in your shoulders, neck, and upper body fully relaxed.

Simple Deep Breathing Exercises

Deep breathing is soothing, relaxing and immensely fulfilling. Given below are some basic deep breathing exercises for beginners.

o **Equal breathing** - To start, inhale for four counts and exhale for similar number of counts. Breathe through the nose. Going to an advanced form, increase the count to six or eight.

o **Abdominal breathing** - Place one hand on the belly and another hand on the chest and breathe deeply through the nose. Make sure that the lungs are stretched as the diaphragm gets inflated with air. Practice six to 10 breaths that are slow for about 10 minutes daily.

o **Alternate nostril technique** - Sit in a comfortable meditative pose, place your right thumb over the right nostril and inhale. It should be deep, once you reach the peak of inhalation, close the left nostril by placing your ring finger and exhale through right nostril. Repeat the pattern from the other side.

o **Skull shining breath** - Begin with a long inhale slowly. Follow it up with a powerful exhale that is generated from your lower belly. Make yourself comfortable with the contraction and stick to one inhale and then exhale. Remember, breath through the nose.

Tranquil Surroundings

Keep surroundings quiet and free from distractions for better attention and focus. Choose a place that is free from noise from the TV or Radio. As and when you practice your meditation skills, you will be able to focus even in areas of high noise levels. You can also achieve this high level of concentration when you continue to practice meditation and strengthen your mind,

Maintain Comfortable Posture

When you are meditating, you must be in a comfortable position. It is only when you are in your most comfortable position that you can get the best out of meditation.

When you have these four elements in place, you can be assured of the best results from your meditation practice.

Get Ready to Meditate

Free yourself from every distraction before you sit down to meditate. These distractions are purely mentally distractions. Meditate during wee hours or before going to bed to ensure tranquility.

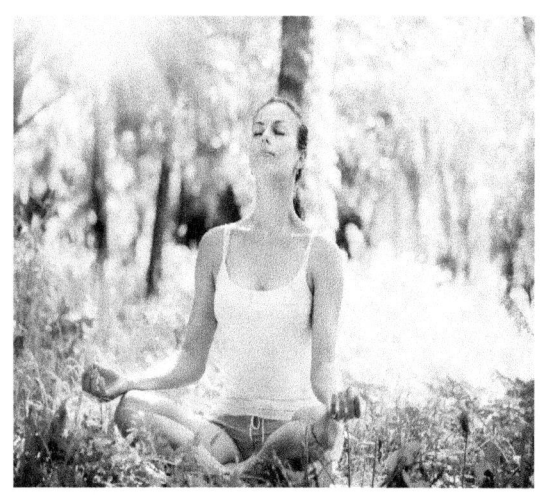

The Suitable Ambiance

In order to meditate, the areas around you must also facilitate it. When you are a beginner, especially, the biggest challenge is getting your thoughts in place and putting all your energy onto one point of focus. The ambiance around you must be one that promotes positive thoughts and complete peace of mind.

If you prefer meditating indoors, there are several things you can do to improve your meditation experience. For instance, you can light aromatic candles to revitalize your senses. For some people, playing slow paced rhythmic music also acts as a great stimulant.

Have a Focal Point
While some prefer to use shrines or statuettes as their point of focus, others like to use a candle to focus their thoughts first and then practice meditating. Several charts are also available to help you focus your thoughts and concentration.

Maintain the Correct Posture
Any position that is comfortable may be chosen to meditate; there are a few

recommended postures that provide maximum benefits. Choose a chair or sit cross-legged on the floor. Keep your spine completely erect. Your life force must be thrust upwards to direct your mind. When you keep your spine straight, you can also avoid pinching of your spinal nerves.

Rest your arms on your thighs. Obtain the Buddha position with your palms placed in the center and facing upwards, or you can place your palm facing upwards on either knee and press your thumb and index finger together.

Your shoulders must be relaxed and rolled back. Relax your neck and keep your chin parallel to the ground. Avoid slouching or leaning forward. You are ready to embark on a divine journey on your own.

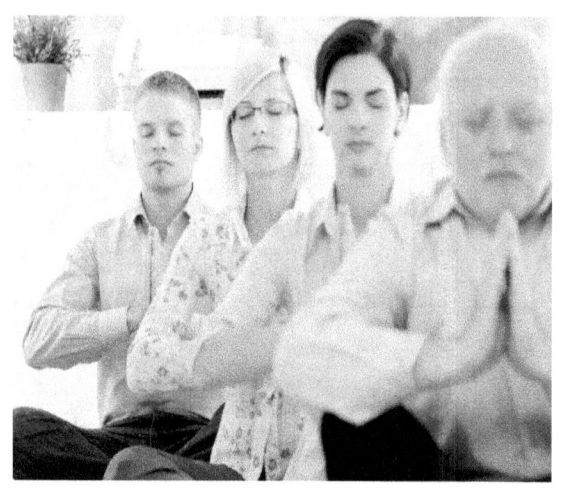

Meditate in a Cohesive Group

As compared to an individual meditating alone, the benefits of meditating in a group are numerous. Meditating in a group will lead to spending more time meditating. We make a bond with others and tend to do what the group is doing.

The energy radiated by many is incredible. It is better when someone provides support and acts as an inspiration to do something. Going for a group meditation is a privilege. There is something powerful about several people channelizing their energy towards one particular thing. There are personal and social benefits of meditating in a group.

Common Goals & Intentions
People who meditate in a group share common intentions. People who get together with a similar intent can have a forceful impact on something. It is simply more satisfying.

Influencing Others
There is a measurable impact on society through people who meditate and some might not even know this. Group mediation will make this practice prevalent with positive results and people will start getting respite from mental unrest and anxiety.

Feeling Mental and Spiritually Connected

On being connected with like-minded people, great impetus gets built up. Even if they are sharing silence and this connection is very powerful. Practicing meditation together will help in getting mutual guidance.

Chapter 4: Meditation Guide For Novices

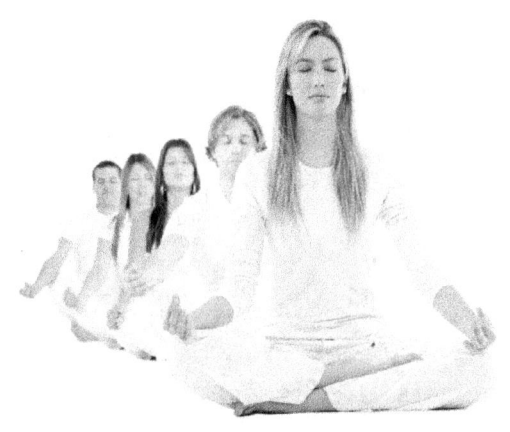

As a novice, there are several techniques of meditation that you can follow. Some of them are ideal for beginners while some may seem extremely advanced for you to get your focus on. For a beginner, the ideal practice would be meditating in a seated posture.

Meditation Techniques

The first challenge is to be able to continue meditating for about 20 minutes without being disturbed. To achieve deep meditation, this is the ideal time.

The idea is to start with 5-10 minutes and then work your way towards longer duration. You can start building on your meditation time only if you find a place that promotes 20 minutes of complete focus. Ideally, sitting in a dark room or a dimly lit room works best for most beginners. Use a timer to keep track of time.

Here are the tips to get you started:

- Set your timer to a convenient length between 5-10 minutes.
- Sit comfortably. Make sure your spine is elongated, and your abdomen is drawn in. Position your hands on lap and take deep breaths. This would relax your anxious mind.

- While breathing out, keep shoulders dropped and relaxed.
- Take two deep breaths before you move on to the next step.
- Now, draw all your focus to your dominant hand. The idea with focusing is to actually feel the dominant hand through your inner eye.

In comparison to any other part of the body, humans are most connected to their physical experiences through their hands. It is through our hands that we can feel and do a lot of things. Therefore, when you are in the earlier stages of your meditation journey, focusing on your hand will able to feel like you are here and now.

Envisioning With Mind's Eyes

• Imagine that your forehead is a window that you are looking out through. Draw you complete attention to the center of your forehead.

• This window leads you to the darkness in your mind. When you tend to look though the window, you will only see darkness initially. This darkness is not permanent. Also, it is never entirely dark.

• Even in this darkness, you will find some amount of light. When you are looking through your inner eye, try to find this light.

• The idea is not to feel the strain that you feel when you are looking at something at a distance. Keep your eyes and your body completely relaxed.

• Just keep looking through the window in your forehead. Then, move back to concentrating on your hands.

- You begin by focusing on your thumb and so on.

- When you switch from looking to feeling, you will have to do two things at a time. While you are focusing on your forehead, you also focus on your hands.

- In the beginning, you will notice you attention shifting between your hands and your forehead. This is perfectly normal.

- Slowly, try to feel both your hands together. This means you focus first on both thumbs and then move to other pairs of your fingers.

It will be easier by joining hands together. When you join your hands, your fingers will touch one another. Nestle your hands in lap to feel relaxed and at ease.

The Challenges

The only problem is that you constantly tend to lose your meditative thought and are thrown back to your aware state. Remember the feeling when you experience your quiet mind state. This feeling makes you feel still and in control of your being. It is almost like a lake on a windless day. When your timer goes off, don't jump right out of your posture. Take your time. Open your eyes slowly and look around the room. Try and understand what you feel as it will be quite different from the time you started.

When you practice these steps regularly, you will be able to achieve a state of deep meditation. This can transform you entirely and improve you as a person. There is no other practice under the sun that has more influence on your being.

Problems likely to be faced are:

Physical Discomfort – Physical discomfort, like pain, is something that is bound to happen in meditation in some form or the other. It is an inevitable aspect of meditation. The purpose should be to eliminate the pain that exists. Physical handling is the key. If you are taking any medication then take it on time so that distractions do not happen during meditation. There can be physical pain while maintaining a posture for meditation but there are remedies to this. Ensure comfortable and loose attire while meditating. In case there is pain in the lower back, then correct the posture. Slouching is uncomfortable, straighten up and do not be rigid. The spine has to be erect at all times while meditating. The hands should be placed in lap comfortably. Neck muscles and arms should not be rigid. Dropping the head forward will cause pain; it has to be aligned with the spine. If still there is pain, then concentrate on it and use it as an object of meditation. Go beyond avoiding the pain and experience the sensation that is below the pain that is being experienced. Pain happens when the muscles are tense around a particular part, try easing and relaxing those muscles and the pain will go away.

Bodily Sensation – Bodily sensation, like numbness, is another problem that happens often when a person is meditating. There is no reason to ponder over this. This happens due to nerve-pinch, and it is not caused by lack of circulation. It causes discomfort but will not cause pain until there is tension caused. One needs to stay calm. Even if the legs go numb and are left that way for the entire meditation period, nothing will happen. It will go away gradually. The body will eventually get used to it through practicing daily.

Strange Feelings - The entire meditation process is different for everyone. There are some people who experience itches, some feel tingling and deep relaxation, there are some who feel light and some feel they are floating. Beginners when experience this get very excited. As one gets accustomed to this, there are sensory signals passed on by the nervous system. This does not mean anything though. One needs just to follow the normal practice as stated above.

Drowsiness - One can feel drowsy during meditation, and it is perfectly normal. Do not get worried about anything like this. This happens because one tends to calm down and relax while meditation and drowsiness will take place. In case of drowsiness, a person should try and focus on drowsiness. Try and locate the feelings and the thought process with drowsiness, and it will evaporate automatically because drowsiness is opposite to inquisitive awareness. Do not eat a large meal and meditate, as this will cause drowsiness. Physical needs of the body like giving adequate rest and sleep is a must; if this is ignored then drowsiness will take place during meditation. In case drowsiness persists, take a deep breath, hold it as long as possible, and slowly release it. Repeat this; it will help sleepiness fade away.

Lack of Concentration - Do not meditate after watching a horror movie or something else as this will hamper concentration. External factors influence the mind and the thought process. Try to meditate first and then plan anything that can influence thought process for the day. Another aspect is the emotional state of the mind. Try resolving daily conflicts as this will reflect in meditation otherwise. Another factor is the state of emotions. In case it is not possible to resolve something important, go ahead, meditate, and do not take this as an excuse of not meditating.

Lethargy and Boredom - It is not easy to sit for a long time, hear the sound of exhale, and inhale. This is bound to cause boredom and should get the treatment it deserves. The steps to treat boredom are reestablishing true mindfulness. Mindfulness cannot be boring and if boredom exists then the practice being followed is incorrect. Correct the practice. Look carefully at the breathing technique being followed and focus technique. They might need a change. Pay attention to the breath. Once a person is mindful of the breath, it cannot be boring. Second is observing the mental state of mind. Pay attention to the feeling of boredom, where is it originating from, why is it happening and what are the mental components of boredom. Once you start looking for the answers, boredom will fade away.

Fright or Fear - People might experience fear during meditation practice, and this has no reason at all. There are many causes behind it. It might be due to something that has been repressed for a long time. May be, if one sits through fear, the cause of fear might erupt and can be dealt with. Everyone who meditates has been or will be through the question that 'What is happening.' It is scary to face the ultimate truth, but someday you will in your meditating process, do not hold back. Just dive deep into it. Another cause of fear is unskillful concentration. The problem is weak mindfulness. The cure to fear is mindfulness.

Anxiety - Agitation happens when the unconscious experiences something deep. Human beings have a habit of escaping something that is not pleasant. Deal with it promptly instead of being troubled by it. The mental energy used to cover-up something remains and keeps causing agitations and distractions. Once you experience this uneasy state while meditating, just observe it, and do not let it dominate. The repressed thought will eventually surface, and you will come to know what you have to deal with. Agitation will pass away if you sit back and watch it.

Trying Too Hard - Take things as they come to you during meditation. Every single day will be different, do not try too hard otherwise, the process will become painful and will not deliver results.

Getting Discouraged - If you try too hard, you will get frustrated, and it will lead to discouragement. Go slow and make note of the progress. Appreciate every single day of the meditation process and discouragement will fade away.

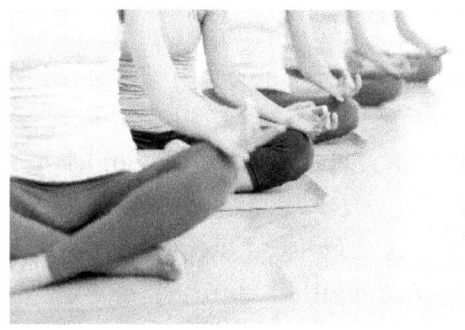

Tips and Suggestions for Beginners

Silence is Pristine

Make sure you choose a quiet corner in your home to make the most of your 20 minutes of focused attention. Your mind must be free from all distractions. This is especially necessary when you are starting off as you have no control on the aware state and the meditative state, and it is usually very easy to snap back. This means that you have to repeat the entire process again and again. This is not only tedious but can also make you lose your patience easily.

Pick Suitable Time

When you are picking your time, make sure that you are never anxious about the next activity. Do not opt for such time spans when the workload in house is the maximum. Else, someone would keep on disturbing you to ask one or the other thing. It is suggested by practitioners that you choose either sunrise or sunset to meditate. This is the time when nature transits from day to night, creating the perfect ambiance for your practice. Plus, the silence at these hours will also add to the tranquility that is a must requisite for the meditation.

Maintain Agility

When you meditate, try to do it just before a meal. If you must eat, then make sure you eat very light before you start your meditation. The reason your stomach must not be too full is that it is very easy to fall asleep during the process of entering the meditative state. When your stomach is light, it makes your mind agiler. Keeping your stomach slightly full will allow you to keep your hunger pangs away. In any case, you must keep small things like hunger in control to make sure you can concentrate completely.

Warming Up

Meditation that is a mental exercise requires a good amount of warming up.

There are simple breathing exercises that you can practice before you move on to meditation. You can start off with some deep breathing. With breathing exercises, you will be able to oxygenate your body completely. Breathing exercises are great at energizing your body and refreshing your senses. You will feel fresh and also extremely ready to focus and concentrate your thoughts to transit from awareness to a meditative state.

Keep Pleasant Demeanor

When you start off your meditative practice, keep a gentle smile on your phase during the whole period of transition. Having a cheerful state of mind will help in meditating in a better way. Don't carry on past incident's bitterness in your mind or the whole purpose of meditation will get defeated. Keeping a cheerful mood will anyways be a better and a preferred way. After all, meditation is for your well-being only.

Be Gentle with Your Eyes

Often, just as people finish their meditation, that they just jump out of their meditative state by opening their eyes immediately. This can ruin all the relaxation that your body and mind have achieved in that time. Even if you have a timer that will go off do not allow it to disturb your state of mind. Make sure you open your eyes gently.

Take Guidance

There are several gurus and teachers who can guide you in this journey. It is recommended that you join a class or find a teacher in the beginning to understand the different methods of meditation. When you meditate without guidance, the disadvantage is that you will find yourself stagnating after a certain period. Those who stay busy, can take help of tapes and CDs that are available to guide you in a step by step process. Taking guidance will certainly give better results as teacher or guide will help in doing the practice in a right way.

Train Your Mind
It is of no use if you meditate everyday but have the rest of your time filled with negative emotions and stress. Enjoy yourself maximum Never expect yourself to jump into a state of meditation if you are unable to enjoy your entire day. You must always create a congenial environment where the meditative state can be achieved easily. Make sure to include activities that bring you joy and happiness even in a mundane routine.

Meditation Techniques

Walking while Meditating - This is a great technique to learn to focus your thoughts. It is a traditional practice that is most suited for people who are highly stressed due to works, emotional trauma or any negative experience. To practice walking meditation, the first thing you must do is find a space outdoors that will keep you undisturbed. Now walk in that space in a slow or medium pace. Keep your entire focus on your feet and on your experiences. Think about positive things that you experience when you walk. Right from the time your toe touches the ground until your entire foot is rested on the ground, the sensations that you experience are quite different. When you observe these sensory details, it becomes very easy to control your mind. The moment you feel your thoughts wandering, you can easily direct them back by focusing on these sensory details. As you practice this, you build your skills of noticing your level of attention and then bringing it back to its maximum. Like this, stay in present and combine a state of physical awareness such as walking with a mental state of meditation.

Imagining Novel Experiences - You must have noticed how something sudden like a leopard crossing the highway suddenly or a policeman stopping your car alters your thinking process. When we experience something new, our brain immediately switches from its day-to-day thoughts and completely focuses on that moment. It is possible to include these feelings even in your daily life. For instance, every time you get back from work, greet your family like you have seen them after a month. You can extend this feeling to all parts of your life including your work. Try to make every task seem like you are a fresher who is enjoying that new experience. Bringing this sense of novelty into every area of your life will help you enjoy your day and thus, improve your meditative practice.

Meditating with Gratitude - Every morning, take two minutes when you wake up to focus before you shift into mundane thoughts like the clothes you are going to wear to work. Think of the people you feel grateful to and all the accomplishments in your life that you are grateful for. Make a silent gesture which is called the 'gratitude signature' to acknowledge that gratitude. Doing this each morning is very useful in helping you invite positivity into your life. Consequently, you will always sit down to meditate, happier and more satisfied.

Chapter 5: Ensuring Effective Meditation

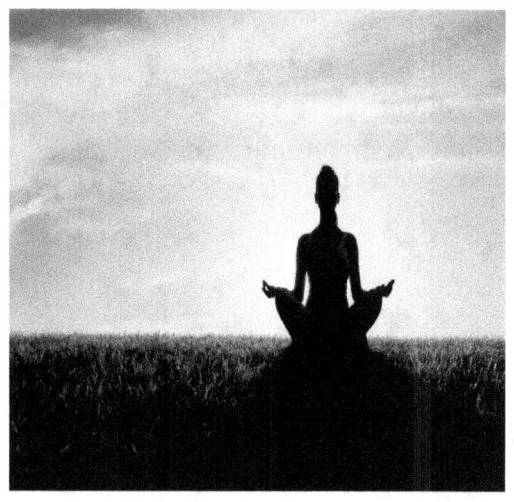

When you start meditation, it is likely that you will feel a little uncomfortable. Sitting in one posture constantly will cause your legs to fall asleep. You may even experience cramps. For those who are practicing walking meditation, feelings of agitation are revived through even paced walking. These experiences may stop, consequently leading to a lot of stress and agitation. The whole goal then becomes experiencing that feeling again causing unreasonable stress. This defeats the entire purpose of meditation.

If such likelihood takes place when you begin to meditate, do not be disappointed or disheartened. It is quite common. You can even try to change your technique of meditation for a few minutes before returning to the normal practice that you are comfortable with. When nothing works, you can try to learn under an experienced teacher who will guide you through these different feelings and experiences.

Expectation from Meditation

Meditation is a practice that takes you through a journey within yourself. You are introduced to physical and spiritual realms that you never knew even existed. Once you have experienced these things, you will see how hard it is to turn away from them or stop experiencing them entirely. Your life will have changed forever after you have these advanced experiences, and the question is if you are ready to comprehend these phenomenal experiences. Your entire perception of reality will change, and you will notice more clarity towards your being that you ever did before. However, it is important to mention here that keeping sudden and rapid expectations from meditation may not be a good idea. Don't expect to feel the tranquility right from the day the meditation is practiced. Meditation is a spiritual practice that will take some time to show its results.

Advanced Stages of Meditation

Experiencing Visions - The first thing that happens to everyone who starts meditating is the experience of certain visions. These visions are indications that you have progressed into a deep state of meditation. Visions occur because the mind has begun opening itself up to spiritual and physical environments. This is only possible when your mind is in a very high state of relaxation. Through visions, you mind adjusts itself to accommodate more advanced experiences.

It is true that your mind need to be rid of several things that hold it back from existing in the high state of efficiency that it is meant to exist in. When you allow your mind to relax, you will see things that may surprise you and bring you back to the state of awareness. As you practice meditation, you will be able to retain that state where your mind clears unwanted thoughts and mental stress.

Spiritual Uplifting - All meditative practices that have sprouted over the years indicate the existence of spiritual guides or guardian angels who watch over us all the time. Many individuals who continue to practice meditation for long periods of time vouch for the solutions and advice that they received from these spiritual teachers or entities. According to Chinese and Japanese ascetics, through meditation, you can achieve a state of mind where you can actually hear the advice that these spiritual teachers give us on a daily basis.

There is a psychological explanation to this process of getting 'answers' and solutions through meditation as well. Through meditation, we clear up all the thoughts and clutter in our mind. These thoughts suppress those areas of our brain that are capable of analyzing the problem and finding solutions. These voices and solutions happen as you move further up your meditative journey. Never try to hear to invoke them or do not try to hear to listen to them. It is natural to achieve higher states of meditation.

Macabre - This experience is only possible when you are at an advanced meditative state. You will be able to sense death through sounds, vision, and even smell, and you will be afraid. These experiences are also of different intensities depending on the individual who is encountering them. These visions of death and experiences of death are not clairvoyant or psychic visions. People often mistake them to be that and give up meditation. When you experience a macabre, you are tapping into that part of your mind that you are afraid of. If you can deal with these fears, you will be completely aware of you existence and will be able to go to the next state of meditation.

Astral Projection - This is a stage that many people are aware of but only a few experience. In the first stage of meditation, we can see visions. In the astral projection state, you can live that vision. You do not merely picture a scene or situation; you can exist in that situation in that brief meditative state. Your mind travels and takes incredible journeys outside your mind and meets new people and visit new places. When you can achieve the stage of astral projection, the control that you gain on your mind is immense. You will discover the endless things that your mind is capable of.

Towards Better Focus during Meditation

In order to move into the advanced state of meditation, you will have to increase your ability to focus and also the time you spend meditating. Like any other exercise, it is necessary to challenge yourself by increasing the challenges in order to get better. To be in complete control of yourself, target the opponents. This process is called targeting.

When you advance in your meditative practices, you will notice that a focus is not merely about thinking really hard about something. When you want to improve your focus, you must try to achieve single-mindedness where nothing gets in the way. When you can attain this state, you will also notice the fact that your energies can be completely channelized to improve your mental and physical capabilities.

Mental Concentration vs. Focus

Making this distinction is extremely necessary if you want to improve your focus genuinely. Mental concentration requires you to hold on to a thought and go over it several times. The result is that you feel a lot more stressed in comparison to being relaxed. When you focus your thought, you allow yourself to look at your thoughts in an unbiased fashion. You would be be able enjoy it from all perspectives and angles. Instead of actually thinking too hard, you allow your mind to find a thought and just indulge in it. Our mind is active at all times. If we are asleep, our mind is still able to perform tasks. This is why we all experience instances when we suddenly find answers to a problem in the middle of a dream. This is the state of focus that you must try to achieve through meditation. Often, we never find solutions to our problems when we are awake because we are constantly trying too hard. When we are sleeping, we never physically focus on getting a solution. We are unfettered by these physical constraints when we are asleep and, that is what focus means.

In order to improve your focus, the idea is to incorporate it into your conscious mind. There are so any things that our sub conscious mind notices but our conscious mind suppresses. This is a defense mechanism from allowing all this information to bombard the thought processes needed on day to day basis.

There is a state of mind called the 'thought- no thought' state when you can focus in a very different way. It is in this state when your body and mind work together to perform tasks. Through this mindset, you allow your mind understand more and see the natural course of action of different things without being limited by prejudices and emotions.

Highly Developed Meditation Practice

When you want to practice advanced meditation, there is a gradual progression that you can work towards. Following tips are suggested to improve your meditation practice:

- Think of the several layers of your mind. There are primal and instinctive parts of your life like food, sleep, swallowing and blinking that make up your existence. Then there is a part of your mind that is pure and innocent.

• It is in this part of your mind that you store all your learning. Try to tap into that part of your brain as it is the most relaxed part of your brain. The other primal part is where all the blocks exist. Your challenge is to reach the state of innocence and heal the other layers of your brain.

• Try to stay awake even through long sessions of meditation. Pay attention your physical health. A healthy body facilitates a healthy mind.

All these techniques require consistent practice and focus. You will have to keep your schedule and incorporate these practices into your daily life to experience the profound impact.

Chapter 6: Meditating During Day To Day Life

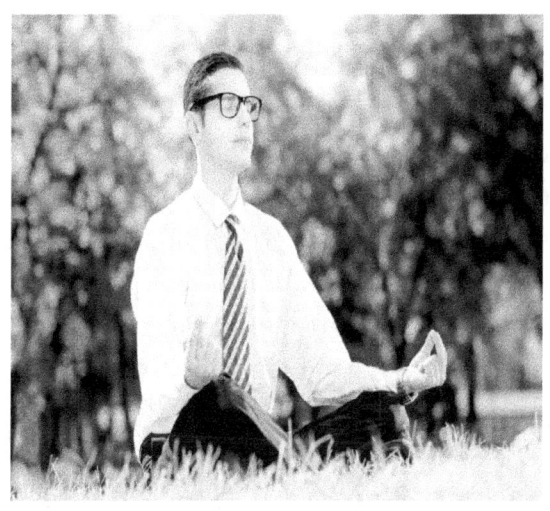

Meditation is an extension of your being. You can incorporate it in all parts of your life and every mundane routine. While you are in control of your thoughts and your actions at all times, you are also able to enjoy even the most boring activity in your life. There are five steps that you can practice every day to make meditation a part of your daily life.

Maintain Level of Motivation - Finding the motivation that you need to meditate is easily the hardest thing to do. To begin with, you can create new meditation environments and use new techniques so that something interesting is there to look forward to each time you start meditation. Get creative when you set that ambiance or environment. Constant motivation is only required when you start meditating. When you begin to experience the benefits of meditation, that itself is good enough to keep you going.

Clarity of Purpose - You must have an intention whenever you meditate. The intention could be as simple as telling yourself that you will make one hour everyday to meditate. You can even have a specifically intended time to meditate.

Self-Realization - There needs to be some agreement that you make with yourself to keep your intentions alive and to stay motivated throughout your meditative practice. You can tell yourself something as simple as "I will make sure I follow my routine for a month, weekends included". Make sure you do not compromise with this agreement because a third party is not involved.

Self-Commitment - No matter what agreement you make with yourself, it is of no use if you are unable to follow through with it. In the beginning, you might find it hard to fight distractions and temptations. However, respect the agreement that you have made with yourself and live up to it as the benefits will be experienced by you in the long run.

Self-Encouragement - Increase your intent as you get comfortable with the one that you have set for yourself. If you are able to sit still for ten minutes of meditation without feeling the stress, then, you can increase the duration by five more minutes to gain momentum. The more you practice, the better you will get. This is how you can gain momentum and get maximum benefits from your meditative practice.

Habitual Meditation

A sedentary position is best recommended for people who have just begun their meditative practice. However, you will notice how easily you can blend meditation into your daily activities. Meditation is only dependent on your state of mind. If you can achieve that state of consciousness through your daily activities, there will be no need to assume a certain position to concentrate and focus.

You can meditate when you are mindful of what you are doing. When you can incorporate mindfulness in your daily life, you will notice that nothing can distract you from meditating. You will be able to meditate at work, in college while shopping and even when you are stuck in a traffic jam.

Mindfulness

The state of being aware of what we are doing is called mindfulness. It is when we apply mindfulness in our daily activities that we can exist at that moment and consequently, meditate in any given situation. The idea of being mindful is not to restrict our mind from wandering. The objective should be to steer away from the thoughts and feelings that occur and gain completely control over when they come and when the leave our mind.

People and machines function almost similarly when it comes to performing tasks. Many activities are to be accomplished in a certain period. However, we are different from machines because all our tasks are associated with emotions and feelings. If the emotions were stripped, we would become mere machines. Unfortunately, the number of tasks that we pack into our daily lives puts us in a state of mechanical existence.

We begin just to drift through our daily activities instead of being fully conscious of what we are doing. We are very seldom aware of the decisions we make, resulting in the loss of clarity in our mind. According to recent studies, close to 50% of our time, when we are performing our daily activities, is caught up in some thought. These thoughts were discovered to be those of confusion and unhappiness.

Try to be mindful off all your experiences. Start with being mindful about the first thing you felt when you saw the line. Then think of the way you are standing. Try to become aware of different physical and mental sensations that you experience in the time that you spend in that line.

Practicing concentration and mindfulness in such situations will help you stay in the present. Then, you will be able to avoid wandering thoughts while meditating in an active state.

Maintaining Consistent Routine

To practice meditation, consistency is the key to success. As you continue to meditate you, develop certain mental muscles like mindfulness and focused awareness. Make sure that you practice meditation on a regular basis. You must also maintain consistency in the quality of meditation and the time you spend. Irrespective of the way you are feeling or the kind of day you have had, make sure you set that time aside in any part of your day to meditate. The only thing you need to do is add an element of focus. You will notice how the most boring and redundant activity will be transformed into a healthy mental exercise.

Chapter 7: Special Meditation Techniques

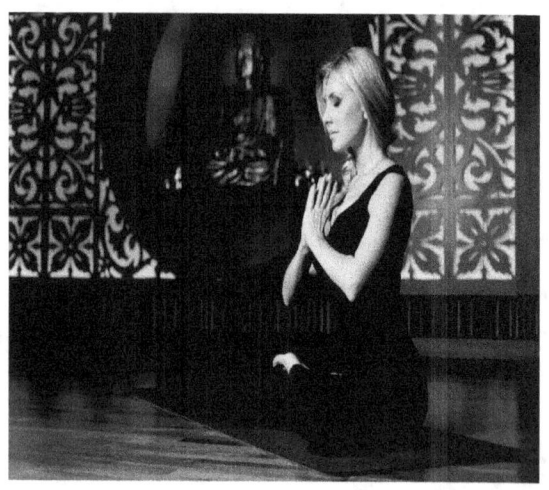

Meditation is not an unknown practice. People have found their meaning of focus and state of meditation. As a result, several techniques of meditation have also been developed over these years. Like we learned before, in Islam and Christianity, meditation is associated with spirituality and devotion. On the other hand, in Asian countries, meditation is based on certain techniques that are designed to achieve the highest possible states of meditation.

When you decide to embark on this journey, you must also be able to understand what to expect. When you choose a guide or a teacher, you must also know what kind of meditation you want to practice. Although it is true that your preferences may change as you progress, it is necessary to know where you want to begin. Here are some well-known techniques of meditation that you can choose from:

Mundane Meditation: We all have some mundane things like cleaning windows or cupboards that we find completely uninteresting. It is a good idea to meditate through these repetitive chores to make them beneficial to your health. For instance, you can count your breaths when you are doing any automatic chore or activity like folding laundry, etc. Since these activities do not require you to be completely attentive and actually make decisions, they are ideal to practice your meditation.

Walking Meditation: This is a type of meditation that is a very enjoyable option. It is recommended by most teachers. When you practice walking meditation, walk consciously taking slow and even paced steps. The point of focus here are your steps. You need not worry about the destination, the distance covered or even the pace, actually. All you need to do is coordinate your steps and your breath. Keep your arms to the side and move them freely. Sometimes trying to control the rhythm of your breath may seem quite awkward. If you feel so, too, just normally breathe and comfortable. All you need to do is be completely involved in the entire process.

Still Meditation: This is a form of meditation that is believed to be very powerful. This type of meditation is capable of building physical, mental and spiritual strength. When you are practicing still meditation, keep your feet apart at shoulder distance. Make sure your knees are soft, and your entire body is relaxed. Your arms need to be placed comfortably on either side. Your entire body must be aligned with shoulders rolled back, an open chest, elongated neck and chin parallel to the ground. Your eyes can be open or must be kept shut very gently.

Lounging Meditation: The classic yogic corpse pose of Savasana is considered ideal for meditation. Lie down on your back with your arms on either side of your body. Allow your feet to fall away from one another. The idea is to keep your body completely relaxed. Although this type of supine meditation is considered to be highly relaxing, the truth is that it makes you stay more alert and also lets you concentrate better. The simple reason is that when you lie down and meditate, the effort that you need to make to stay awake is a lot more. Many people prefer to keep their eyes open in order to avoid falling asleep.

Work out Meditation: This is a great form of meditation that allows you to develop great mental strength while increasing your physical strength. Opt for any form of exercise and convert it into a meditative practice by focusing your mental energy on the physical activity that you are engaged in. There is a certain type of push and pull in your body. Your body also adjusts to new movements that you try. As you work out, notice these small details and you will actually be amazed at yourself.

Breathing Technique: Whenever you need to transit from one mental state to another or from one physical activity to another, this technique is really helpful in making that transition smooth. Take two deep breaths between these activities that you engage in through the day. This practice is extremely effective in incorporating meditation in your daily lives.

Sound Technique: No matter what you are doing, you will be able to notice one repetitive sound that you can focus all your attention on. Whenever you hear the sound that you have chosen to focus on, take two deep breaths. When monks practiced this technique of meditation, they chose sounds like the sound of the temple bell as their centre of focus. The sound that you choose must occur frequently in the setting that you choose to meditate in.

Divine Meditation: The goal of this type of meditation is communicating with God. The idea is to keep calm and focus on the problem in hand. There are mantras or chants that you can repeat to achieve the meditative state that you are aiming at.

People who practice this type of meditation consider is not only highly relaxing but also highly rewarding.

Mindful Meditation: This is the most well known type of meditation. In this type of meditation, you are completely aware of the sights and sounds around you. However, you can bring a sense of fluidity to your mind. You just flow into that state of meditation without focusing on the sounds around you.

Maintaining the Dedication while Meditating

At the time of meditating, the effort that you put in must be correct. There are three elements that you must keep in mind whenever you practice meditation:

Level of Energy: There is a certain law of energy that is associated with meditation. This law states that the more energy you spend, the more you get in return. In meditation, the more wholehearted your effort is, the greater are your returns. There is a limitless source of energy within all of us that you must tap into when you meditate. However, make sure your whole-heartedness does not turn into a struggle. All you need to do is keep your mind relaxed and open.

Earnestness: When you are earnest, you are able to focus better. There will be several feelings and emotions that will tempt you during your meditative practice. You must plug along irrespective of these temptations by holding on to your point of focus. You will notice that day after day, you are able to bring in consistency in your meditation. Earnestness will also put in unique zeal inside your spirit to practice meditation in a better and effective way.

Practice Effortlessness: Don't push too hard to control your mind. When you meditate, you must not do anything that will make you feel too tight and rigid. Do not put in any external effort into your meditation and just allow your mind to surf through your meditative journey.

Chapter 8: Quality Living With Meditation

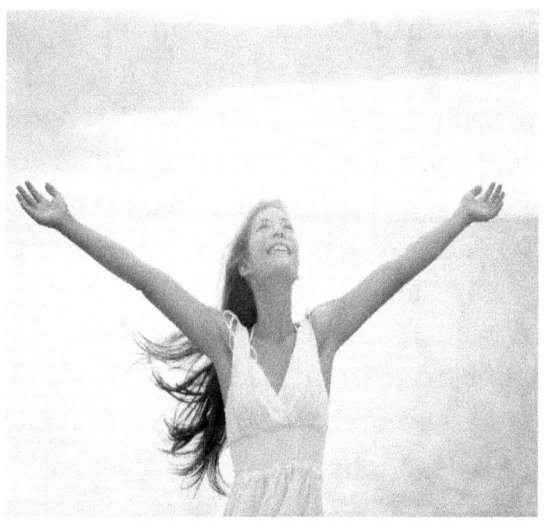

Meditation is one of those practices that are guaranteed to bring about profound changes in your life. As you progress through various stages of meditation, you will notice how simple life itself becomes. Not only are you able to get through boring activities with ease, you will also be able to solve several issues that were only the result of a complicated thinking process.

Researches on Meditation

According to studies conducted recently, meditation has not only psychological effects on us but also has profound physiological impact on us. There is an actual shift that occurs in various involuntary processes of our body and our mind. EEG or electroencephalogram tests showed how effective meditation can be in our life.

An EEG is used to record the mental activity. During physical activities like walking, the EEG readings are actually quite jerky and inconsistent. This shows that the transition of our mind from one thought to another is not consistent. The lines that are recorded are rapid and are known as beta lines. On the contrary, during meditation, the EEG waves that are recorded are an extremely smooth and slow. These waves are categorized as alpha waves. As you move further into a state of meditation, the brain activity becomes slower giving rise to very smooth waves that are known as theta waves.

Research also states that the amount of perspiration is reduced to a large extent. In addition to that, there is a reduction in the amount of metabolic waste found in the blood stream. The immune system gets enhanced and blood pressure gets lowered, according to these studies.

How Meditation Changes your Life

Everyone agrees that meditation is highly beneficial to those who practice it on a regular basis. However, many don't know about the specific ways in which meditation transforms life after a few months of practice. When you start practicing meditation, you will notice the following changes in your own life:

• **Kind heart, mind and soul**

The first thing that you learn through meditation is being kind to yourself. The truth is that it is more important to be compassionate and kind towards yourself before you extend these emotions to other people. Each time you feel like you are having a hard time, you are unable to cope with a situation, are putting yourself down or are unable to deal with yourself, meditation allows you to replace those emotions with kindness. You could be upset, irritated, angry or even struggling to get through certain situations. Then, all you need to do is breathe gently and tell yourself that you will be happy and filled with kindness.

• **Lighter body and high spirits**

Usually the only time we lose touch with inner peace and compassion is when we are stressed. While we are resting, the mind is automatically clear and is able to connect with the deep seated sense of purpose. Meditation is a method that allows you to care for yourself and cure yourself of this negativity. Meditation allows you to spend time with yourself and indulge in the feeling of calmness and thus, lets you cure yourself of an overworked mind. There are signs of stress like your mind getting overwhelmed and your heart closing. This s when you should take some time, focus on your breathing and allow your mind to heal itself.

• **Shedding of ego**

When you can keep that stillness in your thoughts and your mind, you an experience your natural state of being. You can witness all your thoughts and your behavior clearly. This reduces your self-involvement making it easy to let go of the demands that your ego has. You can stop being self-centered and be other-centered, caring about the needs and welfare of others.

- **Dropping of fear and anger**

Our negative thoughts are never easy to accept or release. As a result, we tend to just disown these feelings and simply repress them. However, if our negative emotions lead to shame, anxiety, anger or depression, it is very hard to even repress these feelings. Through meditation, it is possible to actually address these areas of negative feelings and understand how our ignorance towards our negative feelings can also create endless fear and internal drama. Meditation allows you to tap into the quiet stillness that lies beneath this sea of negativity. That is when you actually get to know yourself and experience a wonderful release from you negativity. Practicing meditation for about 20 minutes each day will be sufficient.

- **Learning to be forgiving and compassionate**

Being able to forgive is the most wonderful thing for you and for people around you. Meditation allows you to watch all your thoughts and experience the thoughts that are moving through you. You get to observe the person you really are. You can also see the transition that occurs in you with every passing moment. So this understanding of the transformation helps you realize that the pain caused by another person was, in fact, to a person who is totally different from who you are at this moment. You are able to experience this interconnectedness. Also, you can also get over the separation and suffering that is the result of being unable to forgive.

- **Appreciative and grateful**

Our routine does not allow us to stop and think of the beauty that is all around us. How often do we make an effort to extend our appreciation? When we meditate, the positivity that we are filled with allows us to take a moment and have a sense of gratitude and appreciation for everything and everyone around us.

- **Being aware and mindful**

To feel the sense of inner awakening, it is first necessary for you to become aware. This awareness is inherent in our natural state of existence. Our daily routine is highly reward based. Everything that we do is with the expectation of certain results. However, in meditation, you just do it for yourself. There is no set motive or purpose. So, we do not spend time in the future where we may or may not get that rewards. Instead, we dwell in the present and become completely aware of it. There are no judgments passed or no notions pre conceived. You can enjoy that feeling of being completely aware.

Chapter 9 - Conclusion

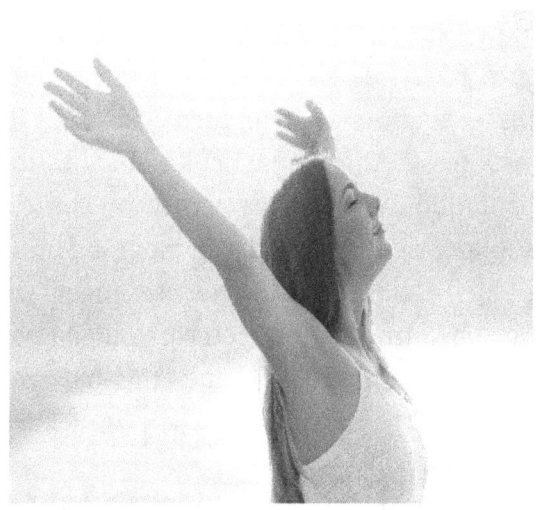

Meditation isn't a new practice. Rather it has been prevalent since time immemorial and evolved through years of understanding and knowledge. Those who have surrendered and acknowledged the power of meditation have experienced its benefits to the optimum level.

Meditation is not a one-day affair; it is an art for a lifetime. Meditation is an art that aligns with the unknown and lets you know the true meaning of life. People have given years and years of their life to this practice and it in turn has done its best to them. A particular meditation technique does not matter, what matters is following it and deriving meaning out if it. Meditation allows you to meet the more beautiful you by letting you go deep into your inner self and making you realize what you are.

Meditation is a state of profound peace when a person reaches a state of tranquility and is fully alert. The practice makes an individual embark upon a journey of inner transformation that makes him reach an advanced echelon of awareness. Meditation is an art that allows people to achieve factual prospective.

Agreed that, most of us may or may not achieve that profound level of self-awareness. However, meditation is the only possible practice that can get us through this amazing, yet incredibly hard journey called life. The focus that we need to get to the purpose of our lives is achieved through meditation alone. Getting over our emotions and being at peace with ourselves not only helps us complete all the expected tasks but also helps us be good at them.